Using Garlic

Planting, Culinary, Medical and Beauty Aspects

By

Gene Ashburner

ISBN-13:978-1502818676
ISBN-10:1502818671

Content

Garlic - Allium Sativum

Scientific Name

Allium Sativum

Family

Amaryllidaceae

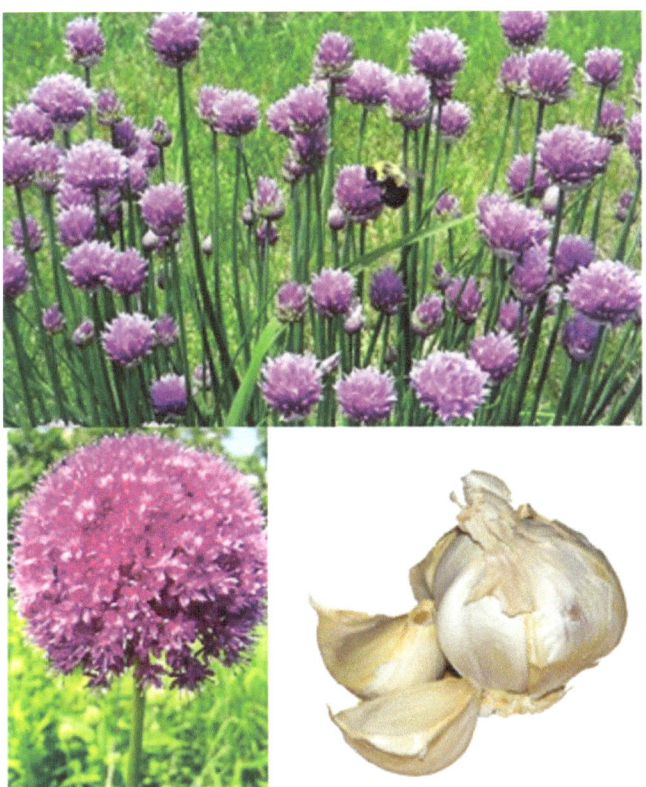

Garlic belongs to the onion family which includes shallots and leeks.

The garlic bulb is divided into sections called cloves.

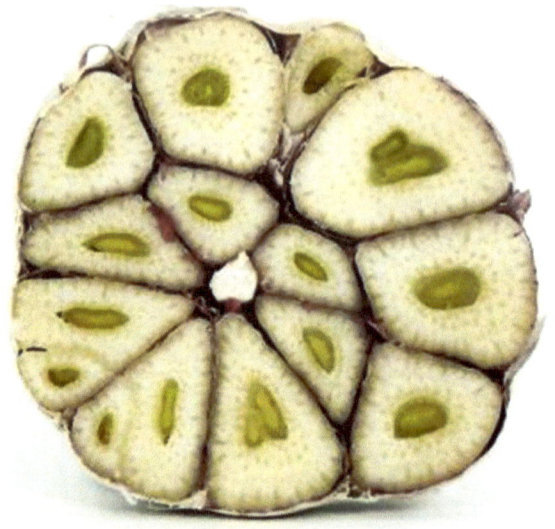

How To Grow Garlic

One garlic bulb has enough cloves to grow an entire vegetable bed full of garlic plants.

Step 1

Fill a pot with good quality potting soil.

Step 2

Split the cloves of garlic apart.

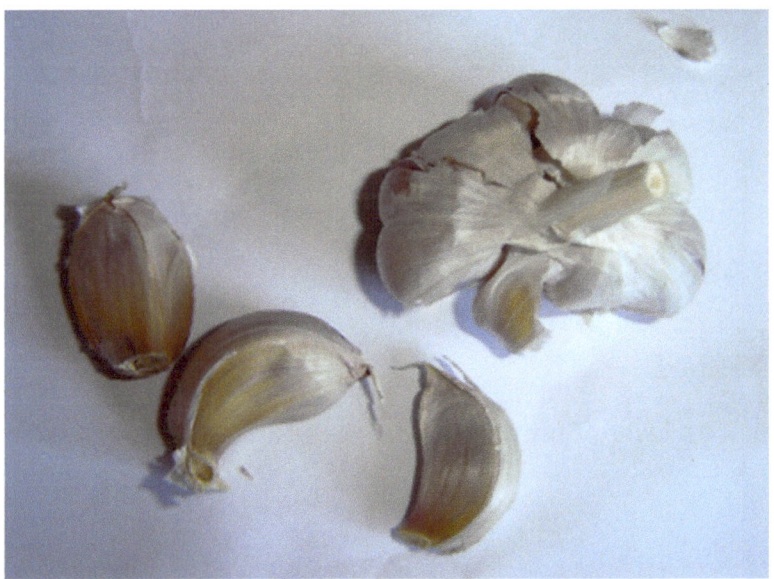

Step 3

Place the cloves of garlic pointy side up in the soil.

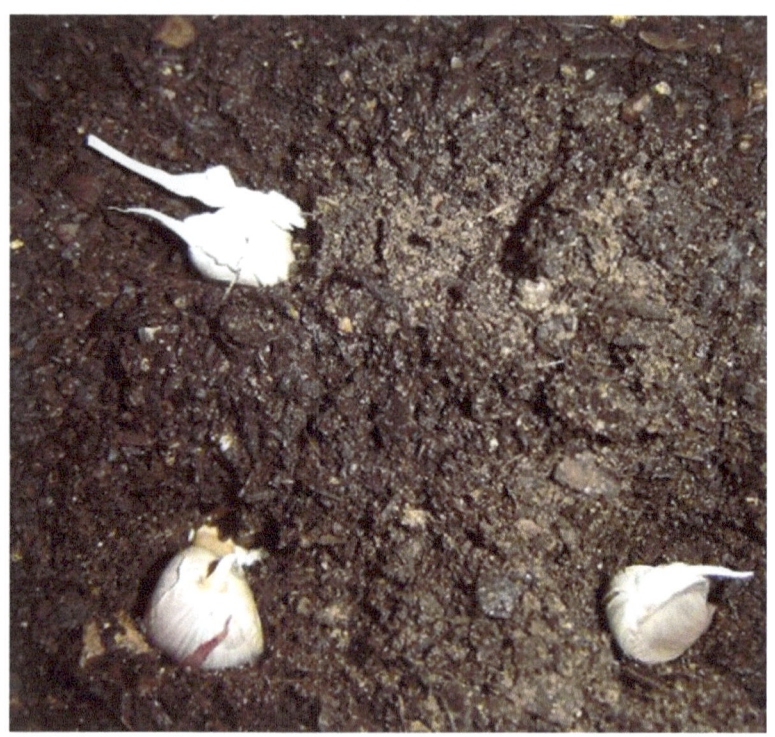

Step 4

Place a layer of potting soil over the garlic cloves.

Step 5

Water the garlic well.

Keep the garlic well watered throughout the plant's lifespan. If you allow the garlic to dry out; the garlic cloves will not swell properly and the garlic will have a short storage life.

Step 6

Place the pot with garlic in a sunny spot.

Types Of Garlic

There Are 2 Types Of Garlic:

Hard Necked Garlic:

- Porcelain, Rocambole and Purple stripe garlic.

Soft-Necked Garlic:

- Artichoke, Silverskin and Creole garlic.

Black Garlic

Black garlic is fermented garlic - whole garlic bulbs are fermented at a high temperature. It is used in Asian cooking.

Black garlic is used as a supplementary food in some countries because of its antioxidants. It is added to energy drinks and garlic chocolate.

Elephant Garlic

Elephant garlic is very large, mild garlic that is more closely related to a leek. This garlic will impart a less pungent taste to the dish you are cooking.

This garlic is also known as Oriental Garlic.

How To Store Garlic

Dry The Garlic

Slice the garlic bulbs into thin slices and place the garlic slices onto a rack. Store the garlic slices at room temperature.

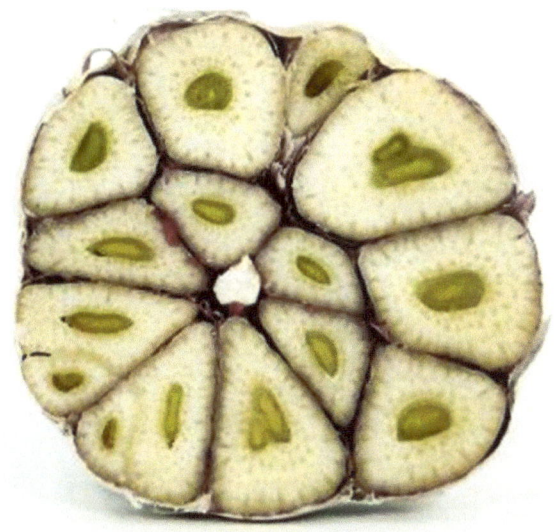

Freeze The Garlic

Freeze the entire garlic bulb.

Braid The Garlic Stalks

Braid the garlic stalks and hang the garlic braid in a cool, dark, place.

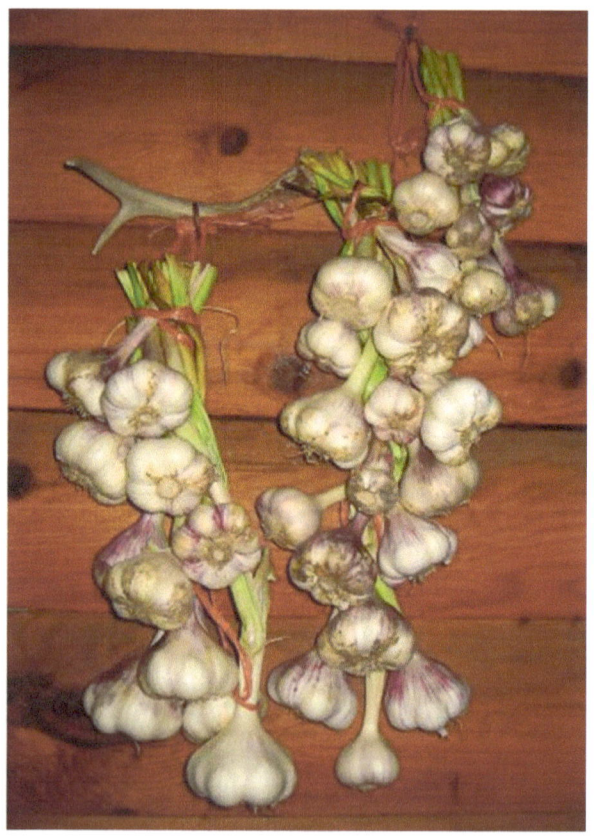

Tip For Storing Garlic:

Garlic will remain fresh for longer if the top part of the bulb remain attached.

Garlic – Different Versions

Garlic Juice – the healthiest way to take in garlic as it still contains Allicin.

Minced raw garlic – also still contains Allicin

Cooked garlic – loses Allicin, not the healthiest way to serve or eat garlic.

Baked garlic – this is a healthier way to take in garlic, cooked garlic loses Allicin.

You can buy garlic bulbs in fresh, frozen, dried and fermented (black garlic) form.

- Dried Garlic flakes
- Dried garlic powder
- Garlic salt
- Granulated garlic
- Dehydrated garlic

Garlic Substitutions

1 fresh clove garlic = 5 ml fresh garlic (chopped)
1 fresh clove garlic = 2,5 ml fresh garlic (minced)
1 fresh clove garlic = 0.5 ml garlic powder
1 fresh clove garlic = 2,5 ml dried garlic flakes
1 fresh clove garlic = 1,25 ml dried powdered garlic
1 fresh clove garlic = 2,5 ml garlic juice

Garlic Used For Culinary Purposes

Garlic is a staple foodstuff in most kitchens and is used for cooking dishes from chicken and pasta to seafood and vegetables.

Garlic always adds a wonderful flavor to the food and a mouth watering aroma to the kitchen.

How To Make Garlic Juice

Ingredients

3 garlic bulbs

Method

Place the garlic into a blender.

Blend until very smooth.

Scrap the garlic puree into a very fine sieve.

Force the garlic puree through the sieve.

Pour the garlic juice into a glass container.

Keep the garlic juice refrigerated.

How To Make Garlic Oil

Ingredients

10 cloves garlic (peeled)
375 ml virgin olive oil

Method

Combine the garlic cloves and olive oil together in a saucepan.

Bring to boiling point.

Reduce the heat.

Simmer for 10 to 15 minutes.

Be careful the garlic does not burn.

Remove from the heat.

Leave the garlic oil to stand for 10 minutes.

Remove the cloves of garlic from the oil.

Slice the garlic cloves.

Spoon the garlic cloves into a glass container.

Pour the olive oil over the garlic slices.

Seal the container.

How To Make Minced Garlic

Ingredients

3 garlic bulbs

Method

Place the garlic into a blender.

Blend until smooth.

Scrap the minced garlic into a glass container.

Keep the minced garlic refrigerated.

How To Roast Garlic

Ingredients

4 garlic bulbs
100 ml olive oil
10 ml sea salt
5 ml ground black pepper

Method

Cut the tops off the garlic bulbs (the top of each clove must be exposed).

Place each garlic bulb into a piece of aluminium foil.

Drizzle with olive oil on top of each garlic bulb.

Sprinkle the sea salt and black pepper over the garlic bulb.

Seal the aluminium foil around the each garlic bulb.

Place the aluminium foil packages onto a baking sheet.

Roast at 400 degrees F for 40 minutes.

Remove the aluminium foil packages from the oven.

Leave to cool on a wire rack.

Recipes

Garlic And Leek Mashed Potatoes

Ingredients

7 potatoes (peeled and cubed)
Salt water to cook potatoes
250 ml leeks (sliced)
12,5 ml olive oil
93 ml cream cheese
93 ml butter
187 ml milk
10 ml minced garlic
10 ml salt
8 ml ground black pepper

Method

Sauté the leeks and olive oil together in a pan until the leeks are soft.

Remove the leeks from the heat.

Set aside.

Combine the potatoes and salt water together in a saucepan.

Bring to boil.

Reduce heat.

Simmer the potatoes until the potatoes are tender (at least 20 minutes).

Remove from the heat.

Drain the potatoes.

Mash the potatoes.

Beat the cream cheese, butter, milk, minced garlic, sautéed leeks, salt and black pepper into the potatoes using an electric beater.

Beat until smooth and creamy.

Garlic And Onion Relish

Ingredients

18 ml olive oil
6 garlic bulbs
2 red onions (unpeeled and cut in half)
5 ml salt
5 ml ground black pepper
15 ml olive oil

Method

Cut the tops off the garlic bulbs (the top of each clove must be exposed).

Pour the olive oil into a baking dish.

Place the garlic bulbs and the onion halves into the baking dish.

Cover the dish with aluminium foil.

Bake at 350 degrees F for 40 minutes.

Remove from the oven.

Leave the onions and garlic mixture to cool.

Peel the onions.

Chop the onions very finely.

Squeeze the garlic pulp from the garlic skins.

Combine the chopped onion and garlic pulp together.

Mix well.

Add the salt, black pepper and olive oil.

Mix well.

Pour the relish into a glass container.

Keep the garlic and onion relish refrigerated.

Garlic Breadsticks

Ingredients

750 ml flour
37,5 ml sugar
5 ml butter
5 ml salt
125 ml cold water
½ yeast cake
Milk
Garlic powder
Dried oregano

Method

Rub the sugar, salt and butter into the flour.

Dissolve the yeast in the water.

Combine the flour mixture and yeast mixture together.

Knead to form stiff dough.

Add milk if the dough is too stiff.

Cover the dough and leave until the dough has doubled in size.

Knead the dough down.

Shape the dough into cigar sized pieces.

Place the pieces onto a greased baking sheet.

Leave the dough to rise until it has doubled in size.

Dust the breadsticks with garlic powder and oregano.

Bake at 375 degrees F for 20 to 25 minutes.

Cool on a wire rack.

Garlic Butter

Ingredients

5 cloves garlic (peeled)
5 ml olive oil
250 ml butter

Method

Combine the garlic and olive oil together in a blender.

Blend until smooth.

Add the butter.

Blend until smooth.

Spoon the garlic butter into a glass container.

Keep the garlic butter refrigerated.

Garlic Chicken

Ingredients

1 chicken (skinned, de-boned and cut into pieces)
250 ml brown sugar
166 ml vinegar
62,5 ml Sprite
37, 5 ml garlic (minced)
25 ml soy sauce
12,5 ml cayenne pepper

Method

Place the chicken in the bottom of a crock-pot.

Mix all the remaining ingredients and pour over the chicken.

Cover the crock-pot and cook on low for 6–8 hours.

Garlic Cheese Dip

Ingredients

1 red onion (peeled ad chopped)
12,5 ml olive oil
25 ml minced fresh garlic
250 ml Gorgonzola cheese (grated)
5 ml ground black pepper
25 ml sour cream
50 ml mayonnaise

Method

Sauté the red onion and olive oil together in a saucepan until the onion has caramelised (about 20 minutes).

Remove from the heat.

Combine the red onion, garlic, Gorgonzola cheese, black pepper, sour cream and mayonnaise together.

Mix well.

Pour into a serving bowl.

Refrigerate until required.

Garlic Dip

Ingredients

2 garlic bulbs (peeled and chopped)
1 red onion (peeled and chopped)
50 ml olive oil
95 ml sour cream
375 ml cream cheese
7,5 ml Worcestershire sauce
7,5 ml mustard
50 ml almonds flakes (toasted and chopped)
20 ml fresh parsley (chopped)
15 ml fresh rosemary (chopped)
7,5 ml salt
5 ml ground black pepper
90 ml cream (whipped)

Method

Sauté the garlic, red onion and olive oil together in a pan for until the onion has softened and the garlic has browned.

Add the sour cream, cream cheese, Worcestershire sauce and mustard.

Mix well.

Add the almonds, parsley, rosemary, salt and black pepper.

Mix well.

Remove from the heat.

Fold the whipped cream into the mixture.

Pour the dip into and bowl and refrigerate until serving.

Garlic Pepper Chicken

Ingredients

6 chicken pieces
37,5 ml garlic sauce
5 ml salt
7,5 ml garlic roasted pepper seasoning
1 can zucchini with tomato sauce
100 ml mozzarella cheese (grated)

Method

Place the chicken in the bottom of a crock-pot.

Sprinkle the garlic sauce, salt and garlic roasted pepper seasoning onto the chicken.

Pour the zucchini over the chicken.

Cover the crock-pot.

Cook on high for 6 hours.

Sprinkle the cheese over the chicken.

Cover the crock-pot.

Reduce the heat.

Cook on low for 30 minutes.

Garlic Pesto

Ingredients

20 garlic scapes
250 ml almonds
374 ml olive oil
125 ml Parmesan cheese (grated)
5 ml salt
4 ml ground black pepper

Method

Combine the garlic scapes and almonds together in a blender.

Blend until smooth.

Add the olive oil.

Blend well.

Add the Parmesan cheese, salt, and black pepper.

Blend well.

Lime And Garlic Salad Dressing

Ingredients

2,5 ml salt
10 ml garlic (minced)
50 ml shallots (finely chopped)
500 ml olive oil
166 ml lime juice
3 ml ground black pepper

Method

Combine the salt, garlic and shallots together.

Add the lime juice.

Whisk well.

Whisk in the olive oil.

Add the black pepper.

Mix well.

Roasted Garlic Relish

Ingredients

4 cloves garlic (roasted, peeled and minced)
10 ml olive oil
12,5 ml lemon juice
3 ml salt
12,5 ml parsley (chopped)
3 ml cayenne pepper
3 ml ground black pepper

Method

Combine the all the ingredients together.

Mix well.

Roasted Garlic Salt

Ingredients

1 head garlic
5 ml olive oil
250 ml sea salt

Method

Drizzle the garlic with olive oil and wrap it in aluminium foil.

Bake at 400 degrees F for 30 to 40 minutes (the garlic cloves should be soft).

Remove the garlic from the oven and allow it to cool.

Squeeze the garlic out of the skin.

Combine the roasted garlic and salt together.

Place the salt and garlic mixture into an oven-proof glass dish.

Bake the salt at 200 degrees F for 20 to 30 minutes to allow the salt to dry out.

Store the roasted garlic salt in an airtight container.

Garlic Used For Medicinal Purposes

Garlic contains many minerals and nutrients and is known to have great medicinal properties as well as antibiotic properties.

This includes the ability to enhance the body's immune cell activity.

The body does not become immune to garlic thus the health benefits will continue over long-term use.

Arthritis Remedy

Ingredients

125 ml olive oil
25 ml minced garlic

Method

Combine the olive oil and minced garlic together.

Mix well.

Apply the garlic mixture to the affected area for pain relief.

Blood Thinning Remedy

Ingredients

   1 clove garlic (peeled)

Method

Eat just 1 clove of garlic per day.

Garlic has a similar effect on the blood as that of aspirin (it will thin the blood).

Bug Bite Remedy

Ingredients

   1 clove garlic (peeled)

Method

Rub garlic onto the affected areas.

The garlic will stop the itching.

Cancer Prevention Remedy

Ingredients

   Garlic

Method

It has been proven that eating garlic daily has a major impact on cancer prevention.

Ear Infection Remedy

Ingredients

1 clove of garlic (peeled)

Method

Wrap the clove of garlic in a piece of tissue paper.

Insert the wrapped garlic into the ear.

Leave overnight.

The garlic will reduce the pain and help fight the infection.

Flu Remedy

Ingredients

1 clove garlic (peeled)

Method

Place the clove of garlic in the mouth.

Bite down every so-often to release the natural garlic juices.

Replace the clove every 4 hours.

Cold symptoms should be gone within 1 to 2 days.

Heart Remedy

Ingredients

1 clove garlic (peeled)

Method

Eat just 1 clove of garlic per day.

This has been proven to be beneficial for the heart.

It will lower the blood pressure, decrease platelet aggregation and lower serum triglycerides and LDL-cholesterol levels.

Hemorrhoids Remedy

Ingredients

Fresh cloves of garlic

Method

Use a pestle and mortar to squeeze all the liquid out of the cloves of garlic.

Apply the garlic juice directly to the hemorrhoids.

You should begin seeing improvements in only one week.

Garlic has proven to have various medicinal properties.

One of these is its ability to treat hemorrhoids.

Herpes Remedy

Ingredients

Garlic cloves (peeled)

Method

Take garlic in 2 ways:

Eat garlic daily.

Rub the garlic clove onto the affected areas.

High Blood Pressure Remedy

Ingredients

Garlic (peeled)

Method

Eat garlic in your food.

Garlic lowers the blood pressure and helps reduce levels of blood clotting.

Iron And Zinc Absorption

Ingredients

Garlic

Method

Eat garlic daily as this increases the absorption of iron and zinc in your body.

Sinus Remedy

Ingredients

Garlic

Method

Eat garlic in your food daily.

Garlic will help clear the sinuses.

Toothache Remedy

Ingredients

1 clove garlic (peeled)

Method

Place the clove of garlic on the aching tooth.

The garlic will reduce the pain.

Wart Removal Remedy

Ingredients

Fresh cloves garlic (peeled)

Method

Rub fresh garlic on and around the warts.

Warts will disappear without a mark with regular applications.

Garlic Used For Beauty Purposes

Acne Remedy

Ingredients

Fresh cloves garlic (peeled)

Method

Rub fresh garlic on and around pimples.

Pimples will disappear without a mark with regular applications.

Antioxidant Remedy

Ingredients

1 clove garlic (preferably aged garlic)

Method

Garlic has a powerful antioxidant effect.

Eat at least 1 clove of garlic per day.

Hair Loss Remedy

Ingredients

250 ml boiling water
25 ml fresh rosemary
7,5 ml garlic juice
18 ml pure honey
18 ml fresh lemon juice

Method

Combine the boiling water and rosemary together.

Leave the rosemary and water to steep for at least 10 minutes.

Strain the rosemary tea.

Combine the rosemary tea, garlic juice, honey and lemon juice together.

Mix well.

Rub the mixture into the scalp.

Leave overnight.

Wash the hair with shampoo and warm water.

Garlic Used For Home Purposes

Garlic Pesticide

Ingredients

500 ml water
50 ml hot sauce
50 ml garlic (minced)

Method

Combine the hot sauce, minced garlic and water together.

Mix well.

Pour the garlic mixture into a spray bottle.

Spray the mixture onto plants to remove caterpillar.

Liquid Garlic Pesticide

Ingredients

Liquid garlic

Method

Pour the liquid garlic into a spray bottle.

Spray the liquid garlic onto plants to keep insects off the plants.

Garlic Used For Pets

Ear Mite Remedy

Ingredients

125 ml olive oil
25 ml minced garlic

Method

Combine the olive oil and minced garlic together.

Mix well.

Insert the garlic mixture into the dog or cat's ear with a dropper.

Garlic And Dieting / Weight Loss

Garlic acts as a natural appetite suppressant.

Garlic contains Vitamin A, C, B1 and B. These vitamins help regulate the metabolism

Best Way To Use Garlic As A Weight Loss Aid

Crushed garlic yields the highest weight lost benefits.

Garlic juice is one of the best ways to consume garlic if you are using it for a weight loss program as it will still contain Allicin. You can either make your own garlic juice – see section Garlic Juice or you can buy pre-packaged garlic juice.

Use garlic raw or baked as these 2 options are healthier than cooked garlic. When garlic is cooked, the Allicin is destroyed. Allicin helps reduce fat levels in the body.

How To Get Rid Of Garlic Breathe

Drink parsley or mint tea to freshen the breathe.

Chew gum that contains Xylitol to freshen the breathe.

Swish your mouth with mouthwash to freshen the breathe.

Swish a little mustard in the mouth, then rinse the mouth with cold water. If the garlic odor is particularly bad then you can also eat a little mustard.

Drink lemon juice to freshen the breathe.

Drink green tea or water to freshen the breathe.

Drink a shot of Vodka to freshen the breathe.

Chew on a sprig of parsley to freshen breathe.

Chew fresh mint leaves to freshen breathe.

Chew coffee beans to freshen breathe.

Sip on milk while eating garlic to prevent the garlic odor afterwards.

Eat cardamom or anise seeds to freshen breathe.

How To Clean A Chopping Board When You Have Chopped Garlic On It

Lemon Wedges:

Cut a lemon into wedges.

Rub the lemon wedges over the chopping board.

Rinse the chopping board with warm water.

Baking Soda:

Combine baking soda and water to form a paste.

Mix well.

Rub the baking soda paste into the chopping board.

Leave for 5 minutes.

Rinse the baking soda off the board with warm water.

www.ingramcontent.com/pod-product-compliance
Lightning Source LLC
Chambersburg PA
CBHW040326010626

45792CB00024B/2167